ISBN: 9798865851769

Beyond Expectations

A father's guide to birth preparation

Alianna Bourgeois

Contents

Becoming Her Partner——————————————————11

Navigating Labor————————————————14
- The Three Phases of Birth
- Birthing Positions
- Pain Management
- Practicing Relaxation Techniques

Pre-Labor

Preparing Together————————————————30

During Labor

Communication In The Delivery Space————————36
- Unspoken Communication
- Becoming Her Advocate

Comfort ______________________________________ 45

• Curating Comfort

Post - Birth

Navigating Postpartum Together ______________ 54

• Systems That'll Save You Time and Energy

• Practical Ways to Show Up

Ready To Support ____________________________ 64

Acknowledgments ____________________________ 69

About The Author ____________________________ 71

Becoming Her Partner

"Commit to the LORD whatever you do, and he will establish your plans."

Proverbs 16:3

When a woman enters into a time of labor, a prepared man helps to keep her grounded and safe. An unprepared man, however, can break her down while she's experiencing one of the most taxing challenges of her life. All praises to the Most High; I had a prepared man for both of my births. Because of his faithfulness to God, his commitment to serving me, and his dedication to becoming knowledgeable on the subject, my husband was the best supporter I could've asked for. Ironically enough, when we first began dating and I mentioned having an unmedicated birth, he was completely against the idea. But as the years went by, he continued to study the nature of birthing with me. As his mind became more familiar with the "who, what, when, where, why, and how," his heart opened up to the concept of a medication-free birth.

For the sake of clarity, this book isn't about birthing preferences. Every woman's situation is different and she has to make a decision that's best for the child's wellbeing, her body, and their coupled safety. Therefore, the point of this book is to walk you through how to be a prepared partner no matter where or how she decides to give birth. As the woman, we're the ones bringing forth this new life into the world. That requires a total submission to God, His plans, His faithfulness, and His ways. Birth, although a physical process, is a highly spiritual act. We need our partners to be our emotional, mental, physical, and spiritual advocates as we endure each phase. We need our partners to encourage us, to protect us from the fears of others and ourselves, to speak truth into us when we're ready to give up, and to be full of discernment to gauge our safety.

Because, although it's physically possible to give birth without a solid partner, it creates unnecessary grief amid a life-changing moment. Avoidable grief that never should've entered into her heart. Birthing is always a wild and complicated ride with potential twists and turns, the last thing that should be added is someone with the capacity to help...but doesn't.

That's why this book is so important to me. For people who can't afford doulas, and even for those who can, there is nothing more special than a man being able to stand in the gap for his partner and fight for her to have a safe and beautiful space to let her body surrender and birth a new generation. Because even the greatest doulas always say that they don't replace the partner, they provide additional support. So, trust in knowing that you're important in this process, more than you may know until the day(s) of.

For the remainder of this book, you'll be introduced to, or reminded of, the various components of pre-labor, labor plus delivery, and post-partum, that you need to be aware of to be properly prepared. I must preface this by saying that this book will not replace essential training from birth workers. Rather, this book is a guide that teaches you what to look for as you two get closer and closer to labor. With that said, let's start your learning journey.

Navigating Labor:
Phases, Positions, And Pain Relief

"Upon You I was cast from birth; You have been my God from my mother's womb."

Psalms 22:10

The Three Phases of Birth

There are three primary phases of birth. Phase one is when she's in early and active labor. Phase two occurs once pushing starts and it ends with the delivery of the baby. Phase three is when it's time to deliver the placenta.

Phase I

The purpose of this stage is to get the baby into the birth canal, aka in position, to be delivered. When you're attending prenatal appointments and they tell you where the baby is positioned, this is why. The first half of this stage is what is called early labor and this could last as long as multiple days or as short as a few hours. Most first-time moms have a longer early labor.

During this time, you'll want to help her balance between resting her body and getting some positive movement to encourage the baby to drop down into the canal. The activities you help her to do will be influenced by the position the baby was in at the most recent prenatal checkup. As she rests, recognize that her body is the freshest it'll be. So, help her to remember not to worry about chores, cooking, etc., and to rest her body instead. One of the easiest ways to advocate for her is to step in and accomplish these tasks so her mind has less to think about. This is also a beautiful time to mentally prepare for the challenges that lie ahead. Take some time to pray, to relax, to bond over entertainment, etc.

It's crucial to stay in close contact with her healthcare provider or midwife during this phase. They can provide guidance and monitor her progress, ensuring everything is proceeding as expected. Keep a record of the frequency and duration of contractions and any other symptoms or changes she experiences. This information will be valuable for her medical team when making decisions about her labor and delivery.

The second part of phase one is called active labor. This is when her contractions will begin to build and her body will begin to experience an increase in pain or surges as some call it. Her contractions will start by being only a few minutes between themselves and this phase usually lasts for up to eight more hours; yet, for some women, this can be an elongated or an extremely short period. You'll want to make sure you're paying close attention to her and not assuming what should be happening based on the classes you take and the information you learn.

The best way to show up for your partner, especially now, is to use your ears more than your brain. Ask her how she's feeling and if there's anything specific she needs. Sometimes, just having someone to talk to or vent her emotions to can provide significant relief. Be her advocate with the medical team, ensuring her birth plan and preferences are respected to the best of their ability. If she needs space, grant it to her humbly. If she needs you to cuddle with her, rest your body with hers. Something my husband did, which I didn't ask of him, was to pray to God before my labor—that he would submit himself to me during my birth. I had never heard of a man praying for such a humble stance before. He told me that it helped him to be in a space of surrender and service so that he could aid me to the best of his ability.

Stay patient and supportive throughout the process. Active labor can be demanding, but your unwavering presence and encouragement will go a long way in helping her through this challenging but rewarding journey of bringing a new life into the world.

Phase II

Phase two is where she enters into what's called the "transition" and ends with delivering the baby for vaginal births. For C-sections, this would be the procedure itself. If she's going through a C-section and you're able to be in the procedure room, make sure to speak life into her throughout the process and to pay attention to things like her oxygen levels, what she's asking for, how she's feeling, etc. Everyone experiences the effects of an epidural differently, and sometimes it can make a woman feel as if she's not able to breathe well, even if she is.

For vaginal births, whether medicated or unmedicated, this can be seen as the homestretch of a marathon. The contestant, aka mom, might be worn out by now and needs some serious encouragement. This is the phase where she might start talking out the side of her neck (meaning crazy) and wondering if she can continue. Be prepared for whatever she says because her bones are shifting, her organs are under pressure, and a literal human is about to come out of her. If she gets short with everyone, don't take it personally. If she gets into a zone and starts to ignore the world, leave her be. If she needs you to recite every encouraging quote you can think of, be ready. This is the shortest phase but it is the most intense. So, when her attitude shifts or her demeanor changes, celebrate because you're getting to the finish line. Finally, don't take lightly the power of being a prayerful partner throughout this process. Take your moments to go regroup, to pray over her and the baby or babies, and to pray over your stamina as well.

The final stage of phase two is the delivery of your daughter(s) and/or son(s). Celebrate the strength given to her, affirm her, and most importantly, bask in the moment. Make sure her providers are still listening to her and that her post-delivery desires are being met (such as delayed clamping, skin-to-skin preferences, etc.).

Phase III

The last phase is the delivery of the placenta. She may opt for medication to help with pain and bleeding, or not. Her body will continue to produce contractions to separate the organ from her body and discard it. This separation will cause her to have internal bodily trauma whether she had a C-section or if it was removed during vaginal birth. The process of delivering the placenta is usually not as intense as delivering the baby itself. The doctor or midwife will keep an eye on things and might gently tug on the umbilical cord or ask you to push a little bit more. Once it's been removed, healthcare providers have to inspect it to make sure it is completely separated. If any part of the placenta is remaining, it will need to be surgically removed as it can cause a deadly infection if not treated quickly. Any portion of the placenta left inside will begin to rot over time and can cause extreme health issues.

I recommend taking her placenta home and disposing of it yourselves. But you can allow the healthcare providers, whether it's the midwife or the hospital doctor, to dispose of it as well. Just know that hospitals, although they have strict protocols with how the placenta is handled, don't have to disclose whether it was discarded as medical waste, or given over for medical research, or even to cosmetic companies.

Birthing Positions

Birthing positions should be based on what feels most natural for her body. Every woman's physicality is different, so forcing her to choose a position that's wildly uncomfortable for her slows down the birthing process. When you take a birthing class together, you'll learn about various positions she can practice standing, laying, or sitting in beforehand. Here are three examples that are most common, aside from laying on one's back.

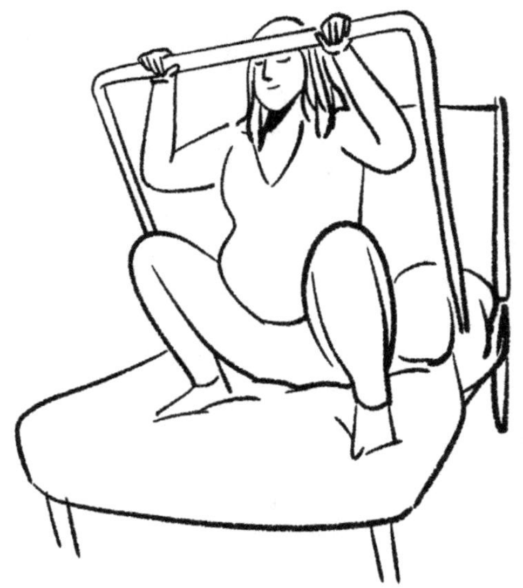

Squatting

To the most ancient of them all, squatting is a position that works with gravity and cuts the amount of time spent pushing. It's a position that's correlated with fewer medical interventions such as the use of forceps while pushing. It's been seen that keeping your feet flat on the ground is also more optimal than squatting while being on your tiptoes. Help her to remember to relax into her heels if she uses this position. You can also help her by putting your arms underneath her armpits while standing behind her to help relieve some of the pressure of this position. However, only do this if someone else is there to help catch baby.

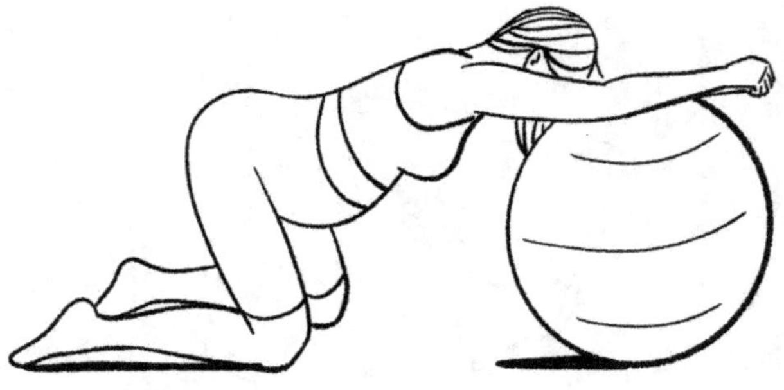

Kneeling

She can kneel in a multitude of ways but the idea is for her to be seated on her knees. Kneeling while leaning over a medicine ball, the bed, etc., can help to relieve some of her back pain if she can withstand being in this position. Imagine your partner being on their knees, similar to how someone might kneel to pray or propose, but in this case, it's to help make the birthing process more comfortable. This position can open up the pelvis and provide a sense of stability and control during labor. It can also make it easier for the birthing person to push when the time comes. As the supportive partner, you can stand beside or behind your partner in this position, offering encouragement, comfort, and any necessary support. It's all about making your partner as comfortable as possible during this important moment.

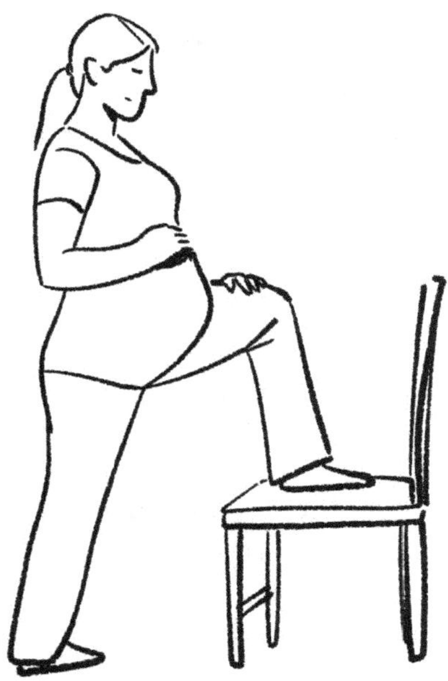

Lunging

If she can stand up and put one foot on top of an elevated object, such as a chair, she can lean her hips into this stretch to help open up her pelvis. She can also use a labor ball underneath her leg to open up her hips more. During positions like this and kneeling, she might favor you to use counterpressure techniques. Imagine it like a sports stance or a deep stretch.

Pain Management

Her pain management preferences should be discussed in advance after she's been able to learn what her options are. You two should also make time to practice the ones that you can do ahead of time to see what her body responds well to. Remember, you might feel helpless when she's encountering this much pain, so call upon your Helper to carry you through while you support her.

If she's in a hospital setting then she'll of course have access to the medications that are offered there. But if she wants to opt-in for a medication-free birth, even if she's at the hospital, remind her of the strength that was built into her body. However, if she's showing signs of failing health, such as a fever, abnormal swellings, excessive blood, etc., move quickly towards safe interventions. And if she ultimately decides to opt-in for medication, even without deteriorating health, make sure to remind her that she's strong and you're standing behind her.

A few non-medication pain management techniques you can consider include:

Water, *nature's epidural*

Water can be incredibly helpful in alleviating pain during childbirth, and understanding why can be beneficial for both partners. Imagine that water acts as a soothing reliever for your partner during labor. Here's why:

Buoyancy: When a person in labor enters a birthing pool or takes a warm bath, the buoyancy of the water helps to support their body weight. This buoyancy can make it easier for your partner to move and change positions, reducing the pressure on their joints and muscles, which can be especially helpful during contractions.

Relaxation: Warm water has a calming effect. It helps to relax muscles and reduce tension. This relaxation can lead to decreased stress and anxiety, which in turn can reduce the perception of pain. Think of it as a warm, comforting embrace from the water.

Pain Gate Theory: Immersing in warm water can stimulate the body's release of endorphins, which are natural painkillers. These endorphins can help block pain signals from reaching the brain, essentially acting as a natural pain gatekeeper.

Hip Squeezes

Hip squeezes can be an effective way to help alleviate pain during childbirth, and understanding why they work can be valuable for the supporting partner. Imagine hip squeezes as a supportive and comforting gesture that can make a significant difference in your partner's comfort during labor. Here's why they help:

Pressure Point Relief: Hip squeezes target specific pressure points located on the sides of the lower back, near the hips. These points are associated with pain relief and relaxation. When you apply firm pressure to these areas, it can help to counteract the discomfort of contractions.

Counterpressure: Contractions during labor can cause intense back pain for some women. Hip squeezes provide counterpressure, which can help relieve this pain by pushing against the pressure created by the uterus contracting. Think of it as a way to push back against the pain and provide some relief.

Support and Connection: Beyond the physical relief, hip squeezes offer emotional support and connection. It's a way for you, as the supporting partner, to actively participate in the birthing process. Your presence and involvement can be reassuring and comforting to your partner during this challenging time.

Distraction: The act of applying hip squeezes can serve as a distraction from the intensity of contractions. It gives your partner something else to focus on and can help redirect her attention away from the pain.

Squeezing Combs

Squeezing a comb is a simple technique that can provide pain relief during childbirth, and understanding why it works can be helpful for the supporting partner. Imagine that squeezing a comb is like a distraction tool in your partner's hand. Here's why it can help:

Distraction and Focus: During labor, the pain can be intense, and it's easy for the person giving birth to become overwhelmed. Squeezing a comb gives them something to focus on other than the pain. It provides a physical and mental task that can help divert their attention and create a sense of control.

Endorphin Release: When your partner squeezes the comb tightly, it can stimulate the release of endorphins like many of the other options listed already. These endorphins can help reduce the perception of pain and create a feeling of well-being.

Tactile Comfort: Holding onto an object like a comb can provide tactile comfort. The sensation of the comb in their hand may create a soothing feeling that helps them cope with the pain of contractions.

Empowerment: Giving your partner something to do, like squeezing a comb, can make them feel more empowered and in control of their labor experience. It's a simple action they can take to manage their discomfort actively.

Breathing Aid: The act of squeezing the comb can sync with your partner's breathing pattern, helping her to maintain a consistent and rhythmic breathing pattern, which is essential for managing pain during labor.

Ice Holds

Holding ice can be a surprisingly effective technique for pain relief during childbirth, and it's helpful for the supporting partner to understand why it works. Here's why holding ice can be beneficial:

Numbing Effect: Ice has a numbing effect on the skin and underlying tissues. When your partner holds ice, it can temporarily reduce the sensation of pain in the area where it's applied. This can be especially helpful if she's experiencing localized discomfort, such as perineal soreness or back pain.

Cooling Sensation: The sensation of cold can be soothing and provide relief during labor. It's like a refreshing break from the intensity of contractions. The coolness of the ice can create a distraction and make her feel more comfortable.

Reducing Swelling: In some cases, holding ice on swollen areas can help reduce swelling, which can contribute to pain relief. For example, if there's swelling in the perineal area, applying ice can help minimize it, leading to less discomfort.

Prepare your mind to remember that the pain that's radiating through her body serves a purpose. Every contraction is not random but rather movement toward an expected end. Constantly affirm her and utilize tools to help her endure.

Practicing Relaxation Techniques

Below is a list of various relaxation techniques, however; the queen of them all is breathing. Breathing is one of the most important tools that your partner has. Attend classes that teach you different techniques to use based on the different phases of labor that she'll be in. Practice them every week leading up to the birth as a moment to center her mind but to also get acquainted with which techniques help her to relax as much as possible. That way, when the main event happens, she won't have to guess which techniques she should use in different moments.

This list isn't an exhaustive one but rather it can be used to spark your all's imagination for the day of. Remember, you can practice everything beforehand. You can create "relaxation date nights," where you test various techniques and see which ones get her in the best state of mind. Here is the list:

1 - Being in the water

2 - Physical intimacy (not limited to sex)

3 - Christian hypnobirthing

4 - Music playlists

5 - Movie lists

6 - Candles and/or incense

7 - Stretching

PRE-LABOR

Preparing Together:
The Importance Of Prenatal Classes

"Be completely humble and gentle; be patient, bearing with one another in love. Make every effort to keep the unity of the Spirit through the bond of peace."

Ephesians 4:2-3

The safest way to walk into unfamiliar territory is to educate yourself on the process, the potential outcomes, etc. So, when I say that prenatal classes are vital in your preparation for her birth, I can't overstate this. Blindly walking into birth with zero idea of what's normal, what's safe, and what's life-threatening, is guaranteed to put you in a disadvantageous position. Education gives you the ability to set your expectations early on for what you can and can't control. What you can and can't do in various circumstances. Where you should and shouldn't go at different phases of labor. What pain you can and can't help mitigate and how. Educating yourself on birth and postpartum could be the difference between you being the rock she needs to endure and the thorn that invokes unnecessary fear.

According to my husband, prenatal classes were more beneficial than he originally thought they would be. In the beginning, he saw the classes as if they were for me and he was just there to support me by being present. This is a common idea held by men about prenatal classes. You might be thinking of these sessions as something that's for her and won't help you in many ways. However, that's the furthest from the truth. Prenatal classes are for both of you, not just her. There is so much information you'll learn that'll teach you how to tend to her and even how she's thinking about this journey.

And because my husband is the head of our household, he used the prenatal classes as an opportunity to know how he would be submitting unto me during my labor to ensure my safety, comfort, and confidence. If reading that made you uncomfortable, go and study Ephesians 5:21. Continuing: by participating in the classes and learning what I would physically be going through, it helped him to better understand what I may have spiritually needed. This gave him the sensitivity and awareness not to take anything personally, to set the tone of my birthing space, and so much more.

As his wife, him attending those classes with me increased my confidence and trust in him. I can't get myself pregnant, so it wouldn't be fair if I was the only party actively preparing to birth our child. His presence showed me that he was taking full responsibility for this new life even before we got to hold them. Gratefully, our classes were hosted by our doula whom we have a great relationship with, so both of us were comfortable and eager to learn. Reflecting on that journey, we engrossed ourselves with as many opportunities to learn about birth as possible. We would stay up and watch birthing videos on YouTube, so when my time came, neither one of us would be thrown off by all of the bodily changes, release of liquids, emotional outbursts, etc. I wanted us to be as prepared as we could possibly be.

So, what is a prenatal class? This definition can be found on Pregnancy, Birth, and Baby's website, "Antenatal classes are also called labour and birthing classes. They help you get ready for labour, birth, breastfeeding, and caring for a newborn baby."[1] A few things you should expect out of your prenatal classes:

- **Increased Confidence in Birth Awareness:** Prenatal classes offer a comprehensive understanding of the entire birthing process. You'll learn about the stages of labor, what to expect during each phase, and how to recognize signs of progress. This knowledge will boost your confidence, allowing you to be more actively involved in supporting your partner during labor. When you can anticipate what's happening, you'll be better equipped to provide comfort and reassurance.

- **Preparedness for Unexpected Turns:** Childbirth doesn't always go as planned, and unexpected complications or changes can arise. Prenatal classes help you prepare for such situations by discussing potential challenges and alternative birth scenarios. This knowledge empowers you to adapt to changing circumstances and make informed decisions alongside your partner.

---

1   https://www.pregnancybirthbaby.org.au/antenatal-classes#:~:text=Antenatal%20classes%20are%20also%20called,them%20along%20to%20the%20classes.

- **Understanding Pain Management Interventions:** Prenatal classes delve into various pain management options available during labor, from natural techniques like breathing exercises and massage to medical interventions such as epidurals or nitrous oxide. Understanding these interventions allows you to support your partner in making informed choices that align with her preferences and comfort.

- **Awareness of Medications:** Prenatal classes educate you about medications that may be administered during labor, including their benefits, risks, and potential side effects. Knowing the options enables you to engage in meaningful discussions with your partner and healthcare providers, helping you both make informed decisions about pain relief and medical interventions.

- **Confidence in Birth Planning:** Your partner's birth plan is a crucial component of her childbirth experience. Prenatal classes equip you with the knowledge and confidence to fully understand and support her birth plan. This includes advocating for her preferences, communicating effectively with the medical team, and ensuring that her wishes are respected to the extent possible.

But the only way to gauge whether or not the class is of any benefit to you two is to be mentally present during the sessions. You can't test if you're learning anything if you're not trying to learn anything.

If you're working with an OBGYN and/or a doula, they'll have recommendations for classes you can attend if they don't host them themselves. If you don't have access to any provider at the moment, 'YouTube University' is your best friend. You'll want to make sure you learn about these topics:

- **Her birthing anatomy**
- **Stages of labor**
- **Common complications and various solutions**
- **Positions of the baby**
- **How to progress labor**
- **Pain management techniques**
- **Pain management medications**
- **Emergency protocols**
- **Breathing techniques**
- **Pushing techniques**
- **Nutrition during labor**
- **Delivery bag items**
- **Baby's post-birth exam**
- **Breast and formula-feeding techniques**
- **Postpartum care, healing, and expectations**

Prenatal classes are going to be a huge benefit to you as the one partnering alongside her. You'll be able to intimately learn about the ins and outs of birth which will allow you to help her craft together a birthing plan that makes her feel secure. So, go into these classes with an open mind and know it's just as much for you as it is for her.

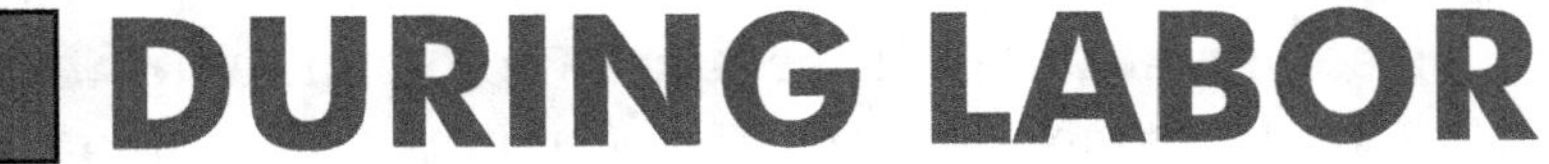

DURING LABOR

Communication and Advocacy In The Delivery Space

Romans 14:19

This portion of the book will go through various topics you'll want to consider during the labor. This chapter will specifically touch on communication and advocacy. These topics, although not medically related to birthing, have a huge impact on the quality and speed that birthing takes place. I believe this is because communication and advocacy both open up the opportunity for safety and security to co-exist. And when the woman's body feels safe, it responds more readily to all of the internal birthing cues that encourage it to move along. However, when it doesn't feel safe, it does all that it can to hold baby on the inside until the threat, whether real or perceived, has been removed.

Let's begin with talking through open communication and how it evolves over the course of labor. For most, open communication during labor is communication that frees her from having to worry about how she's communicating at that moment. The way she speaks during this time might be wildly different than how she speaks on a random Tuesday with no contraction pain. Although it may seem silly to describe it this way, it'll be a useful reminder for you. Her pelvis is currently expanding to make room for another human's head, or sometimes feet, to come out. The way she asks you to bring her water or relief might be drastically different.

Although I'm not advocating for women to become monsters to those who are there to help them, I think we need to be honest and accept that immense pain can shift how we communicate with others. Looking back over my births, I can pinpoint how my communication styles shifted depending on which phase of labor I was in. I was the most talkative during early labor. This makes sense given early labor is when our body is the freshest it'll be in this process. For the most part, this is when we'll still feel most like ourselves and can clearly articulate our different needs. For me, as active labor progressed, I had fewer words and relied on my husband to know me and my body well enough to help me even when I lacked the ability to speak.

Having that space to just speak freely helped me to stay focused on the mission at hand—birthing baby. All of my emotional processing was focused on how my body was doing, where the baby was inside of my body, etc. If my husband didn't allow this space, I wouldn't have had as much liberty to focus on what was going on internally. Imagine going through the worst pain of your life and worrying about how you might sound when you're trying to communicate what you need. But with the security of my husband, I didn't have to think about what I had to say, how to say it, or whether my words were sweet or sour, because he created space within himself to take them and help me. Again, this isn't justifying a woman verbally assaulting her team and telling everyone how awful they are, but rather, allowing her to communicate what she needs without worrying about how she's being perceived. So, her yelling, "Get out of the room!" isn't taken negatively.

Unspoken Communication

As the contractions ramp up in both speed, duration, and intensity, she's going to likely use fewer and fewer words. However, this doesn't mean she's communicating with you less. Once her body begins to fatigue from laboring, she'll begin to use unspoken communication, aka nonverbal communication.

Relational intimacy is the only way to understand what her body is communicating to you without her explicitly saying it. And although sex is a way to learn about her body, this isn't what I'm referring to when I say relational intimacy. As she's living her life, how does her body look? How does her body express sadness? What about joy? What faces does she make when she's overwhelmed? How about when she's hungry? It's your job to pay attention to her in such a way that by the time you make it to labor, you can help her even when she doesn't have the energy to tell you what's going on. Being able to see her in this way keeps you from over-asking and potentially underestimating how much pain she's going through.

My husband was able to read my face and know I was becoming frustrated. He could tell how I was moving my body when the waves of the contractions were hitting or coming to a close. He knew when I needed to get more water, take a bite of a snack, etc. He wouldn't have been able to see these needs if he hadn't taken the time to pay attention to me. While I washed the dishes, how I carried myself after a rough day at work, the way my face shifted when my song came on...these seemingly small details gave him a framework for who I am and how I move.

Now, how are you supposed to use all of this information? It's not to have a memory bank of random information. Instead, your goal during labor should be to reflect on her patterns and use that to encourage her. God is her sustainer, but trust that He's going to use you to help her stay motivated to endure. How you communicate, verbally and nonverbally, has immense power in the birthing space. If she's asking for something and you don't help her in a timely manner, if she says something in a tone you don't like and now you have an attitude, you could stir up feelings of loneliness, fear, rejection, anger, etc., in her that prolong the birth. Now, instead of focusing on helping get the baby down into the right position, her mind is on you two, which keeps her from doing what she needs in that moment.

Spaces that don't feel safe always, and I do mean always, prolong birth. This isn't good for her or the baby because each of them is combatting the exhaustion for longer periods, increasing the danger of complications. With this in mind, be aware of your attitude, your expectations, your word choice, etc. Use your body, your actions, and your words to affirm her in the strength of God and how He will see her through. You don't have to tell her you understand what she's going through, because you don't, but you can demonstrate that you're grateful for her endurance and commitment to seeing this through whether via unmedicated birth, medicated birth, or C-section.

Becoming Her Advocate

Now that you're thinking through communication styles and how to pay attention to her nonverbal cues as well, it's time for us to cover advocacy. This topic is near to me because proper advocacy can legitimately save a woman's life. So, first things first, I want you to think of advocacy as protecting and serving, not just cheerleading. When she goes into labor, even if you've been through birthing with her before, neither of you knows how she's going to respond. And in the case that she physically, mentally, and/or emotionally shuts down, you need to be the one that ensures she's receiving proper care. You have to know what she deserves and desires because if she shuts down, it's not her job to ensure she's being treated well. With that said, she'll always remember how you protected or neglected her during this time. Trust me, just because you're not having the baby doesn't mean you don't have a very pivotal role in this process.

Something our doula taught my husband and I was how when a lioness goes into labor, the lions stand outside of the den where she's located to make sure nothing gets inside to disturb her. If in the chance that they neglect to protect a particular area and another animal invades her birthing space, the labor could extend for days or even weeks until a safe space has been re-established. The lions' standing guard is a perfect example of what advocacy looks like. No one wants to be giving birth while having to stay on the defense the entire time. Everything about labor and birth is an extremely offensive play that requires large amounts of focus and concentration.

In practicality then, what does advocacy look like? In my opinion, it starts by knowing and respecting her birth plan. You won't know what boundaries are being tested or potentially crossed if you don't know the boundaries and expectations that have already been set. The best way to know these plans is to also be a part of the creation process. Your role isn't to dictate to her what should be happening in her plan, but rather, to allow her to dictate to you what makes her feel secure and how she expects things to flow in emergencies. Because everything she knows about this plan, you should know too. You want to be aware of every nook and cranny. For example, my husband knew that I didn't want a space where people felt comfortable to bring their worries. I needed to be protected from their opinions while I undertook one of the hardest things I've ever done in my life. So on the day of my first birth, he pulled our mothers aside and reminded them not to allow themselves to spill out their worries over me, and if they became overwhelmed to use a different part of the house to decompress. He also gave them different tasks like doing the laundry, cooking us food, etc. And at one point he could see on my face that I was beginning to feel overwhelmed so he asked everyone to leave the room. I didn't have to ask him because he knew in great detail what I needed and wanted out of my birthing space. He knew that his role was to protect me and provide me with my needs first and once those were taken care of, provide me with my wants. My needs were safety, hydration, communicating with others on my behalf, etc. My wants were the lighting in the room, music playing, and so on.

What can advocacy look like then? In a medical environment, advocacy could look like reminding the staff that she's allowed to walk around and labor instead of just laying in the bed if she and the baby(ies) are doing well. It could look like reminding the midwife that she declined to use any form of intervention to progress labor. To make it plain, advocacy is willingly standing up on behalf of another. It'll require you to be willing to mean what you say while staying gentle with the people you're speaking to. You can help direct them while keeping the peace. Remember that everyone, including the doctors, is here to support and serve her. She isn't at the knee of anyone here.

I realized we've talked about advocacy for a second now and I could ramble about this subject for days because I feel so protected by my husband. But if you know you struggled with protecting her in the past, know you can do something different now. There's always an opportunity for growth. Affirm to her that you want to become a better nurturer of her body and her soul. To summarize this point, here are some points you can quickly return to as a reference:

- **Ensuring Her Wishes Are Respected:** By advocating for your wife, you're ensuring that her birth plan and preferences are communicated clearly to the medical team. This helps create an environment where her choices are respected, and her voice is heard. Your advocacy ensures that she doesn't feel pressured into decisions that don't align with her wishes.

- **Providing Emotional Support:** Labor can be emotionally challenging, and your presence as an advocate offers emotional stability. You're there to provide encouragement, reassurance, and a comforting presence throughout the process. Your support can ease her anxiety and make her feel safer and more secure.

- **Effective Communication:** Advocacy often involves effective communication between you, your wife, and the healthcare providers. You help bridge any communication gaps by ensuring that questions are asked and answered, information is shared clearly, and decisions are made collectively. This collaborative approach ensures that everyone is on the same page regarding her care.

- **Supporting Informed Decision-Making:** Advocacy means being well-informed about the various aspects of labor and delivery. By understanding the available options, risks, and benefits, you can assist your wife in making informed decisions that prioritize her health and the well-being of the baby. This partnership in decision-making is a fundamental aspect of advocacy.

- **Being Her Voice:** In moments of pain or vulnerability, your wife may find it challenging to advocate for herself. Your role as an advocate means being her voice when she needs it most. Whether it's expressing her preferences or concerns or seeking clarification from medical professionals, you ensure that her needs and questions are addressed.

- **Creating a Supportive Environment:** Your advocacy contributes to the creation of a supportive and empowering birth environment. This not only helps your wife feel more comfortable and in control but also fosters a positive birth experience that she can look back on with satisfaction and pride.

Comfort:
Techniques For Labor Relaxation

"Blessed be the God and Father of our Lord Christ, the Father of mercies and God of all comfort, who comforts us in all our affliction, so that we may be able to comfort those who are in any affliction, with the comfort with which we ourselves are comforted by God."

2 Corinthians 1:3-4

This chapter is about relaxation techniques. In our everyday lives, we don't tend to think of relaxation as a practice but rather as a state of being. But one of the benefits of experiencing birth two times is learning that relaxation requires action and can be created even in the toughest situations. My doula introduced us to a range of various techniques that I'll be sharing in this chapter. No matter what stage of pregnancy your partner might be in, it's never too late or too early to begin practicing these methods together.

The goal of relaxation techniques is to help train her mind to regulate itself despite the intense waves her body is experiencing. These techniques aren't to resolve the pain, instead, they should be used as a tool to aid in her endurance. If you're familiar with any long-distance sport, then you've likely heard of gels. Gels were created for athletes to consume while performing to give them a new boost of energy for their muscles. The gels never take away the pain associated with the activity. They simply supply nutrients that allow the athletes to keep on going. So, when choosing techniques, you want to remember that these are for relief but they will never, especially during active labor, remove the pain entirely.

Remember how birthing positions are dependent on the woman and her preferences? It's the same thing for relaxation methods. While I'm laboring, I have to stay in constant movement. I would pace, sway, and work on breathing low. If I needed a second to recoup, I would lead over the couch, the bed, etc., anything that would still allow me to rock my body while resting. I tried the peanut ball, laying down, etc., and those methods didn't work for me at all. But, that doesn't mean those techniques weren't useful; they just didn't work for me, my anatomy, and my preference. While researching, I recommend you all compile a list of ten different techniques you can begin practicing. Below, I'm going to highlight five different types and different things you'll want to consider as the supporting partner.

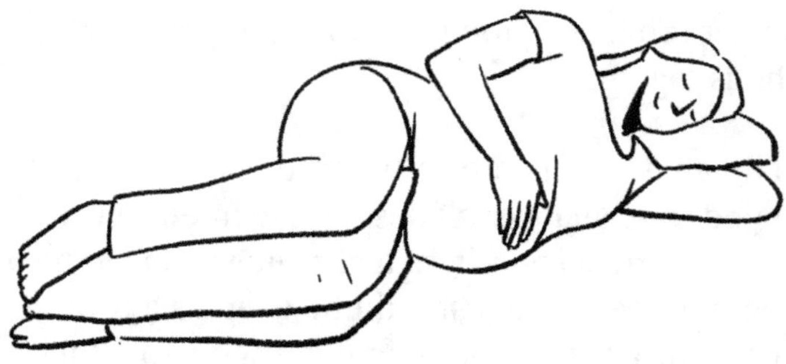

Deep Breathing

When your partner practices controlled breathing, it enables her to remain calm and composed, even as contractions intensify. Slow, low, and steady breathing will also save her so much energy and force her to focus her breaths during contractions. As the pain increases, she will have a stronger desire to become more high-pitched in her breathing, potentially resulting in yelling. When you hear her pitch getting higher, gently remind her to "bring herself back down," and "to keep it low." Labor is an energy game, and I don't mean it in a good vibes kind of way. I mean it in a marathon run kind of way. The more we can focus our actions, the less energy we're burning unnecessarily, and the more we'll have in the tank to keep going.

Visualization

Setting her eyes on the Kingdom of God will keep her in ways that I can't even fully describe. There is something about thinking about the goodness of God while being in the midst of something that's crushing us that brings an unexplainable peace. You can help her with this by speaking the Word of God over her, by reminding her of the promises of the Kingdom when she's feeling helpless, and by being in private prayer for her during labor.

Counting

This is exactly what it sounds like. Think of this method as counting sheep but instead of for sleep, it's used as a distraction from contraction pain. Someone somewhere said that the brain can't focus on two thoughts at once (try it), so the idea is to replace thinking about pain with numbers. You can support her with counting by counting out loud with or for her. One way you can practice counting is for you to call out the odd numbers while she calls out the even numbers. Note that you should count at a tempo that allows her to keep a slow, low, and steady breath.

Progressive Muscle Relaxation

Also denoted as PMR[2], this has been clinically shown to help reduce stress and anxiety. The protocol is as follows; you will select a muscle group to focus on by tightening and then relaxing. Follow this example: Clench your jaw for three seconds, then slowly release for two seconds. You will choose a different muscle group to do this with until you've covered your entire body. This technique requires some focused practice to become aware of your different muscle groups and how to individually activate them, so encourage her to give this a few tries before deciding if it's helpful or not. You can support her here by doing a few different things. First, calling out the muscle groups for her and counting her down. Second, gently poking the area she's meant to be tensing up to help bring her awareness to that area. Third, you can follow along with her.

---

2   https://www.cci.health.wa.gov.au/-/media/CCI/Mental-Health-Professionals/Panic/
    Panic---Information-Sheets/Panic-Information-Sheet---05---Progressive-Muscle-Re-
    laxation.pdf

Physical Support

This is a broad way of labeling different ways that you can use your body to help relax. You can study options like counter-pressure, back rubs, gentle touch, etc. Just make sure that you remain mindful of her and use the sort of touch that helps her feel safe. Also, she might not want physical contact at all and that's both normal and okay. Your goal is to be a sort of aid for her whether that means being close or at a distance.

Remember, your job now is to find ten different relaxation techniques to practice over time and see which ones she enjoys the most. Once you know which ones seem to work the best, write them down so you have them handy for game day, aka labor.

Curating Comfort

As you all practice your list of ten relaxation techniques before narrowing down which ones she prefers, I want you to also consider the environment. An environment that's been crafted for comfort can truly change the way she experiences her birth. This is one of the top reasons women are opting for birth centers or birthing from home. The ability to create an experience that's customized down to the lighting of the room, the smells, etc., is something you can curate; even if she's opted in for a hospital birth.

My husband talked about how providing comfort for me was like being my cheerleader. And although he wasn't stereotypically high tempo, loud, or even super verbal, he was consistent in his encouragement, his comfort, and keeping me grounded as my partner. He stayed in the Spirit so he could keep me fueled. He knew that my experiences would be unique, as it is for each woman, and he constantly asked for the Lord to provide me with strength, and that I would look to the Almighty for endurance. And based on his own experience with training his body and his mind, he kept at the forefront of his mind that the body can last longer than our thoughts communicate to us. But that ability to press on comes directly from God.

So, spiritually, I was extremely covered, which gave me an internal comfort to know that I had someone warring for me even in the moments I didn't have it in me to war for myself. But that's not where he stopped. He also took it upon himself to make sure that my environment was comfortable for me physically. While I was washing my mind over with scripture and trying to keep my eyes toward heaven, he was considering my hydration, my food intake, the music I wanted, where people were in proximity to me, etc. These might sound like small tasks but by him heading them out, I could sit with the pain I was experiencing and communicate to myself that although the pain is real, God is with me through it all. Even if I were to lose my life in this, I'd be with the one that's kept my soul.

His focus on my overall state of comfort also gave me space to think rationally during the moments when we had to pivot our original plans. For example, after my firstborn was delivered, I had an extreme tear during delivery that sent us to the hospital. Once we got there, I was rushed into surgery and my husband had to take care of our newborn by himself. A newborn that was ready to feed. I can't tell you why, but the hospital didn't have any pacifiers for him. Now, considering the comfort of our child, my husband created a makeshift pacifier to get him through the two hour long surgery until he could nurse with me again.

I can't overemphasize how necessary my husband was in the experience I had with my birth, and my prayer is that as you go through this guide, you see how many ways you'll be able to step up and be an active participant in this experience. And although it is a lot of work, it's work the Lord is willing to help you walk through. So, yes, consider refreshments, snacks, pillows, lighting, temperature, music, anything that can create a beautifully sacred and protected space for her, whether you're her romantic partner or not, because this child(ren) deserve to be birthed in a space where the womb they're exiting was well taken care of.

To bring it down to practicality, these smaller miscellaneous things such as food, temp, etc. should be discussed before she's 37 weeks ideally. Even better, make sure to order everything that's shelf-stable or non-food related by the time she's 36 weeks, so you can have her bags packed and ready.

POST-BIRTH

Navigating Postpartum Together

Welcome to the fourth trimester aka postpartum, the phase that occurs once there is no longer a baby inside of her womb. The only catch to this trimester is that it lasts far longer than three months. You can look at it physically where it's a year or more of true recovery after birth let alone emotionally. You're healing from 9 to 10 months of carrying a child, typically, and then the intense and internally traumatizing process of delivering this child whether vaginally or the extreme surgery of a C-section. And for the mamas that experienced loss, now you're healing from the process of growing a child you won't get to know on this side of heaven. This stage, by far, tends to be the most taxing. A child has left your womb. An internal organ has ripped itself apart from inside of you, aka the placenta. It's a beautifully scary time that will require you to have an immense amount of empathy, care, and of course, patience.

This is where your protective care kicks it up. The way you curated her environment during birth doesn't stop at the end of delivery, it evolves and continues into the next phase of her healing. Because now all of those hormones that made her womb suitable for that new life are going haywire again to readjust to her sole anatomy. These same hormones impacted her hair, her teeth, her ligaments, her tendons, her fat stores, etc. Plus, if she's breastfeeding, the rollercoaster of her hormones increases times ten. And to top it all off, the very structure of her brain has changed after all of this. I'm not writing this to paint her like a beast, but instead, I hope you're accepting that this next phase isn't a return to normal. Matter of fact, it's the establishment of an entirely new way of being. She needs you to protect her environment so she can heal. Imagine the kind of care you would need if someone ripped an organ out of your body if your pelvis expanded itself, or if someone cut through your skin, your fat layers, your muscles, and into an organ to take just one part of it out. You would, rightfully so, be down for a hot second. For later reference, here is a list of miscellaneous facts surrounding the postpartum period:

- **Postpartum Recovery Duration:** The postpartum period typically lasts around six weeks, but full recovery may take longer for some women.

- **Perineal Discomfort:** Up to 95% of women experience perineal discomfort, including soreness and pain, after vaginal childbirth.

- **Cesarean Section Rates:** Approximately 1-in-3 births in the United States is delivered via cesarean section (C-section), and recovery after a C-section can be longer and more challenging.

- **Postpartum Mood Disorders:** Postpartum depression affects around 1-in-7 women, making it essential to be aware of the signs and symptoms.

- **Breastfeeding Rates:** In the first few weeks postpartum, nearly 80% of new mothers attempt breastfeeding, which can be a physically and emotionally demanding process.

- **Sleep Deprivation:** New mothers often experience sleep deprivation, with most getting less than five hours of continuous sleep per night during the early postpartum weeks.

- **Fatigue and Exhaustion:** Nearly all new mothers report experiencing fatigue and exhaustion, which can have a significant impact on their physical and emotional well-being.

- **Hormonal Changes:** Hormonal fluctuations after childbirth can lead to mood swings, night sweats, and other physical and emotional changes.

- **Physical Recovery:** It can take several weeks for the uterus to return to its pre-pregnancy size, and pelvic floor muscles may require time to heal.

- **Support and Emotional Well-being:** Emotional support from partners and loved ones is crucial during the postpartum phase, as feelings of isolation and anxiety are common.

- **Return to Work:** Many women return to work within twelve weeks postpartum, which can be challenging as they juggle work responsibilities and childcare.

- **Body Image Concerns:** A significant number of women may experience body image concerns and pressure to "bounce back" to their pre-pregnancy appearance.

- **Sexual Activity:** Resuming sexual activity can take time and communication between partners, as physical and emotional factors play a role in postpartum sexual health.

- **Contraception:** Postpartum contraception is an important consideration, with some methods recommended to begin soon after childbirth to prevent unintended pregnancies.

- **Self-Care:** Encouraging self-care for the new mom, including rest, proper nutrition, and relaxation, is essential for a smooth recovery.

Systems That'll Save You Time and Energy

Before getting to the postpartum phase, spend some time considering all of the things that keep the home running. Here are some starter questions:

- How often do we do laundry?
- How frequently do we clean and put away the dishes?

- How often do we cook or buy food?
- What days of the month do we have bills due?
- How often do we need to clean the bathrooms, bedrooms, etc.?
- How much do we typically spend per week?
- Who's usually in charge of what at the house?
- What are our work schedules?

By assessing what's going on already and considering all the new changes that are on their way, you can begin to prepare systems that'll help you two out when you're in the thick of a sleep regression running on two and a half hours of sleep. We didn't implement this technique I'm about to introduce during my first postpartum phase, but during my second, I practiced what is referred to as the 5 by 5 by 5. This protocol has the mother spend five weeks in bed, five weeks on the bed, and five weeks around the bed. Essentially, it's a way for her to ease back into the swing of life by confining her to the bed, then in the bedroom, and finally with activities that can be done close enough to get back in the bed if necessary.

Jeremi and I both agree that we wish we had heard of this for the first go around. Not only did it give me proper time to get through the initial start of healing, but it also helped to temper expectations around when I'd start moving around again. By knowing this, we knew at minimum how much time we'd need extra hands to help around with cooking, cleaning, laundry, etc., especially while my husband was at work and I was on leave, then before I went back to work and he took his leave.

Practical Ways to Show Up

Calling Your Community

It's pretty common for the mother to call on her community to come help during this phase. But rest assured, you can call on yours too. Your homeboys more than likely shouldn't be over at the house the way her homegirls would be, but they can still pitch in. You'll need help to help her too. Ask them to put in grocery orders and have them drop them off. Let them know your all's favorite food spots and ask if they can get you a gift card there. Tell them about the size of diapers you know you'll need in the near future. Have them stock up on wipes. But at the top of the list, talk to them about what you're going through and ask them for prayer and encouragement. Serving her and this new child will require you to die to your flesh, and you'll need healthy support, especially from other men, to refuel you.

Preparing Your Finances

If you're reading this book and there's still ample time before the baby's anticipated due date, think of ways you can save money here and there or make additional cash to be used during the postpartum period. You can have someone come out to deep clean the home towards the tail end of the pregnancy and again around three months postpartum. You can save up for premade meals that are high in protein and fiber for you two to help keep your bodies nourished. You could also save up for fun times where you can send her out on a quick date with herself, you two can go out for a mocktail or two, go see your favorite DJ, or whatever reminds you of the bond you two have despite all the responsibilities that have to get done day to day.

Get Domestic

Brother, one of the biggest stressors on her mind during this period will likely be keeping up the home. It doesn't matter if you're on leave with her, if you're working a full-time job, etc., put your hand to the plow and help around the house. There is a beautiful humility, honor, and respect that comes with helping take care of the very home God called the two of you to steward. And in the postpartum phase, you'll likely need to take on more than you would in the past to keep things flowing. A clean physical space will also give her the emotional space to tend to you, herself, the baby, and other children you all may have. She is one of your greatest investments in this life; honor her by being willing to lead out in domestic household duties.

Create Your Outlets

The first being you should run to for strength, energy, etc., is the Most High. Let reading your Bible, prayer, and worship be your daily anchors. As you prioritize these, also create some sort of schedule that keeps your body moving, your hands creating, your mind thinking, and your heart laughing. Ask trusted family members to come tend to her and the home while you go see your family and friends. Or, ask someone to come help while you get some alone time. If you want, you can use this weekly and monthly structure to plug and play for yourself. The activities could be done in five or sixty-five minutes. Don't tell yourself you can't simply because you think you need to dedicate a ton of time to each of these.

Daily - God time

Three times a week - Move your body

Once a week - Push your mind (learning)

Twice a month - Use your hands

Once a month - Go laugh with yourself, family, and/or friends

Outlets remind us that we're whole beings and we're needy. God created us this way and it allows us to constantly look to Him for our strength and to lean on our communities. Forcing yourself to do everything alone eventually not only hurts you, but it'll hurt your family. Because mom and the kid(s) are best when you're healthy spiritually, emotionally, mentally, etc. With that said, this period can bring out some of the worst in ourselves. Make sure that you're paying attention to her and yourself for constant feelings of extreme anger, sadness, or doom. Look online for postpartum depression and anxiety screenings you two can take every few weeks if she doesn't have a midwife to report to after birth. You should also consider finding a faith-based therapist ahead of time, in case you want to start individual therapy at this time.

Before concluding, here's an extended list of ways to show up for her post-delivery:

- **Cook Her Favorite Meals:** Surprise her with homemade meals she loves. Preparing nutritious and delicious food can make a significant difference, especially when she's adjusting to the demands of motherhood.

- **Take Over Baby Duties:** Offer to handle night-time feedings or diaper changes, allowing her to get some much-needed uninterrupted sleep. Even one night of good rest can do wonders.

- **Create a Relaxing Bath Time:** Set up a soothing bath with candles, music, and bath salts. This can provide her with a peaceful escape and a chance to unwind while you take care of the baby.

- **Plan a Spa Day at Home:** Arrange a spa day at home with massages, facials, or foot rubs. You can even hire a professional masseuse for an extra treat.

- **Coordinate a Postpartum Photographer:** Capture those precious early moments with a postpartum photoshoot. It's a wonderful way to celebrate her strength and the new addition to your family.

- **Write Love Notes:** Leave small love notes in unexpected places, like in her wallet, on the bathroom mirror, or tucked into a book she's reading. These gestures can remind her of your love and appreciation.

- **Host a "New Mom Retreat":** Organize a day where she can pamper herself with friends. Invite some of her closest friends over for a spa day, coffee, or just some quality time.

- **Learn Baby Massage Techniques:** Take the time to learn baby massage techniques together. This not only benefits the baby but also creates a bonding experience for both of you.

- **Surprise Date Nights at Home:** Plan surprise date nights at home after the baby is asleep. Cook a special dinner, watch a movie, or enjoy a board game together.

- **Plan a Weekend Getaway:** If circumstances allow, plan a weekend getaway for just the two of you, even if it's a short stay at a nearby bed and breakfast. It can be a refreshing break from the daily routine.

- **Create a Memory Book:** Compile photos, mementos, and notes to create a memory book of the pregnancy and birth journey. It's a beautiful way to preserve these special moments.

- **Offer a Listening Ear:** Be there to listen and provide emotional support. Sometimes, all she needs is someone to talk to about her experiences and feelings.

Expect everything to change whether in a minor or a major way, and seek the Lord to have peace in it. Because she's becoming an entirely new woman, you're becoming a new man, and it's all for your sanctification and the glory of God. Relearn her and yourself, and pay attention to new desires and patterns of thinking. And by all means, never cease praying for your household.

Ready To Support:
A Final Recap On Your Birth Partner Journey

"And my God will supply every need of yours according to his riches in glory in Christ."

Philippians 4:19

My prayer for you is that you will take this guide and the information that's inside of it, and take action. Whether you can or can't afford a doula, OBGYN, midwife, etc., doesn't determine the way you can show up and be a necessary part of this journey. Here's a mini checklist you can use to make sure you're on the right track. You don't have to do everything on this list, specifically, if you already have a solution.

- Search for and hire a doula and/or midwife if possible

- Find an online course created by a doula and/or midwife if you can't hire one at the moment

- Study unmedicated births at home, a center, or a hospital

- Study medicated births at a center or a hospital

- Find birth plan PDFs that she can use to create her own birth plan

- Learn about the hospitals that are closest to you in case of an emergency

- Watch calm live births together

- Learn about pain management techniques

- Learn about pain management medications offered in hospital settings or with a midwife

- Find a simple exercise regimen for her that prioritizes getting the baby in position

- Consider how your community can help during postpartum and start sharing your desires with them ASAP

- Talk about your expectations of each other come postpartum

- Create a savings goal and account for the postpartum period

- Start looking into individual therapists for each of you

- Create a list of easy but fun things the two of you can do after baby is born

- Talk through which family members or friends the two of you trust to help with baby (remember, a decision like this takes two yeses and only one no)

- Think through outlets that move your spirit, body, mind, hands, and heart

The information you've read through is your starting point for a whole world of knowledge ahead, but you are capable of learning it, retaining it, and most importantly, utilizing it. Lean into the servant leadership role you've been called to and trust that you won't feel capable all of the time, but God's grace is sufficient for you. Be willing to listen to her, to the professionals you either hired or studied online, and of course, God. Put on the Spirit of Christ and be a true servant and advocate for her. Humble yourself while she's walking through one of the most humbling experiences of her life. She needs you, even if she doesn't know how to properly articulate that, and so does this new life.

With that being said, Congratulations on embarking on this incredible journey of fatherhood! Your desire to show up as the best partner for your wife after she's given birth is truly commendable. Remember that in this new chapter, your love and support can be a source of immense strength.

The postpartum period can be both joyous and challenging, and your role is crucial. Be present, be patient, and be understanding. Your wife has just given birth, and her body and emotions are adjusting. Your unwavering support, a listening ear, and a comforting presence can make all the difference.

Stay proactive but also adaptable. Be willing to take on new responsibilities, whether it's changing diapers, preparing meals, or offering to give her a break when she needs it. Every small gesture counts. Know that it's okay to seek help and advice when needed. Parenting doesn't come with a manual, and it's perfectly normal to have questions. Reach out to other experienced fathers, healthcare professionals, or parenting groups for guidance and reassurance.

Celebrate the small victories and cherish the precious moments. From the first smile to the late-night cuddles, these are the moments that create lasting memories. Above all, remember that your love and dedication are the greatest gifts you can offer. You are embarking on a journey filled with love, challenges, and growth. Embrace it with an open heart, and you will become the best partner and father you aspire to be.

Your wife and your new baby are incredibly lucky to have you by their side. Believe in yourself, trust in your love, and enjoy every moment of this remarkable adventure.

Peace and blessings.

Acknowledgments

Thank you to my husband for supporting me throughout our marriage and in particular, this project. Thank you, Kiah, for being my partner in this huge and transformative time in my life. I also want to acknowledge our moms, Maria and Kinta, for being so strong and open to unmedicated birth, and for being such pillars on that day. My birth team, Ashley, Eve, and Carmen, thank you for changing my life and the lives of so many others. May The Most High God bless you all, and your works.

About The Author

A proud mother of two, whose journey into the world of birthing began with two successful home births that transformed her life. Her incredible husband's unwavering support during those labor moments ignited a passion within her to empower birthing partners. Guided by her faith in Christ and the surrender of herself to God, Alianna stared fearlessly into the face of childbirth, embracing its beauty and wonder. Now, she is on a mission to create a guide for birthing partners, sharing the transformative power of love, faith, and support during the incredible journey of birth.

www.ingramcontent.com/pod-product-compliance
Lightning Source LLC
Chambersburg PA
CBHW060802260726

48660CB00002B/734